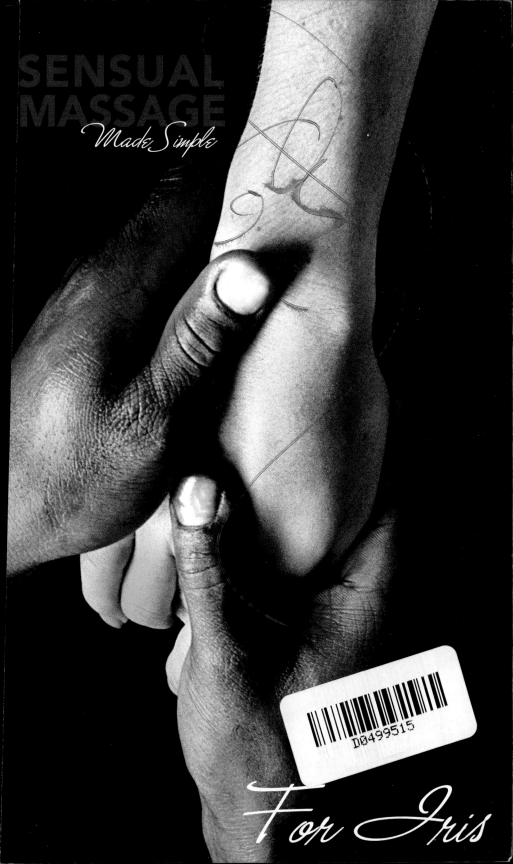

First Printing—September 2008

Always consult a doctor if you are in doubt about a medical condition.

ISBN 978-0-9748535-6-7
Library of Congress Control Number: 2008902743

Printed in China

an Arcata Arts book
arcata-arts.com

TABLE OF CONTENTS

Tips, Master Strokes 4

Chest 13

Head 25

Arms 37

Hands 49

Feet 61

Front of the Legs 73

Back 85

Back of the Legs 97

Specialties 109

Repeat most massage strokes three times—
more if your partner moans with pleasure.
Be generous during a massage.

MASSAGE TIPS

- Choose a warm (at least 70° F/21° C) quiet place.
- Be generous with cushions and pillows.
- Make room to move. Look after children and pets.
- Trim and file your fingernails, wash your hands.
- Dim the lights, play your partner's favorite music.
- Turn phones off. Never rush.
- During rotations, move three times in one direction, then reverse. Repeat kneading strokes at least three times.
- During percussion, cover an area three times.
- Repeat circulation strokes on the arms and legs ten times.

Blend your oiling into the strokes you are doing while maintaining a consistent rhythm.

OILING

- Oiling makes every massage movement (except friction and percussion) easier.
- Oil every part of the body except the scalp and eyelids.
- Add a few drops of lemon to a light oil like safflower or walnut.
- Warm your oil before starting. A plastic squeeze bottle will prevent spills. A flat-based bowl works too.
- Warm your hands before oiling.
- Add oil to your hands, never pour it onto your partner's body. Oiling marks the beginning of massage. Be silent. Let your hands say it.

Use light pressure just below the ribs where the lower portion of the kidneys are exposed.

- Transitions become opportunities to extend a sensual moment.
- This stroke moves from the back of the knee to the thighs and lower back. Maintain contact at the knee and ankle throughout. Avoid jerky motions.

Get feedback on pressure if it's a first massage, but don't encourage conversation.

Kneading travels well; use it on every fleshy part of the body.

- Move your hands in opposing circles. Lift a fold of flesh and squeeze gently with one hand, while releasing with the other. Knead with your fingertips on the hands and feet. Use the full surface of your hand on the back, legs and sides.

At the beginning of all circulation strokes, press toward the heart.

CIRCULATION

• Start at the ankles, making contact from the tips of your fingers to the base of your palms.

• Push forward over the legs, back and shoulders, molding your hands to the shape of your partner's body.

Rotate the fingertips of your right hand, the friction hand, on the muscles below. Friction converts the uninitiated to the pleasures of massage.

FRICTION

• Press down until you feel solid muscle; avoid bony areas and surface blood vessels. Keep your fingers together.

• Steady the body with an "anchor hand" (here, the left hand). Friction strokes spread a tangible warmth.

Percussion sets up irresistible waves of sensation that penetrate deep within. No oil is necessary.

- Always modulate the "blows" by relaxing ("breaking") your wrist or tapping on the back of your hand. Create a spreading vibration. Concentrate on visible muscles.
- Get feedback from your partner on what feels best.

You do all the work,
your partner does
nothing at all.

PASSIVE EXERCISE

- Passive exercise increases the body's mobility.
- The body provides convenient natural "handles" at the wrist, ankles, chin, shoulders and lower back.
- Use them to lift and flex the joints. Gentle pressures will do.

11

Compression works almost everywhere on the body—and it always feels good.

COMPRESSION

- Compression is the easiest massage stroke.
- Simply fold one hand over your wrist and press down evenly from the knuckles to the forearm. Circle slowly.
- Make contact from your fingertips to the base of your palm.

CHEST

Slowly move your anchor hand across the chest. Follow with the friction hand rotating in small circles.

FRICTION

- Anchor the chest with one hand while rotating on the full, flat surface of your fingers. Press harder on muscular tissues.
- On bony surfaces flatten your friction hand to spread the pressure. Vary the pressure as your rotate.

Hold for a moment at the top of the lift, then lower your partner slowly.

BODY LIFT

- Reach through the hollow of your partner's back and lace your fingers together over the spine.
- Lift with the full surface of your hands, spreading pressure evenly. Maintain an even rhythm while lifting and lowering.

15

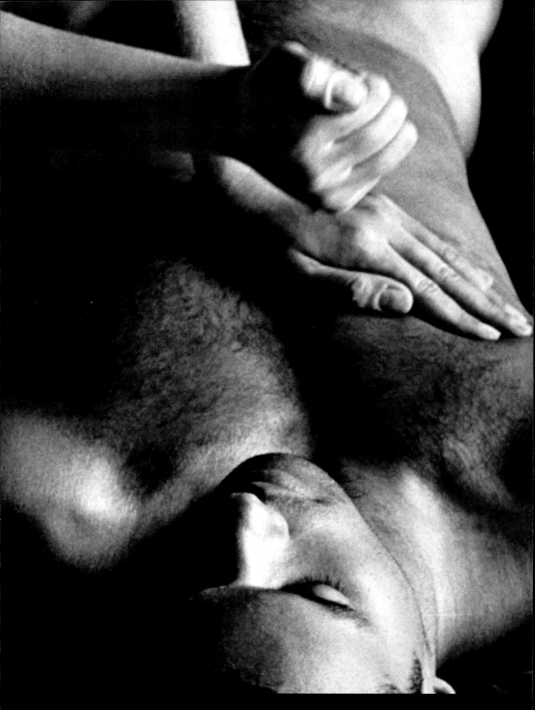

POUNDING

- Tap the top of your closed fingers with the side of your fist. Relax (or "break") your wrist as you make contact.
- Move your closed fingers back and forth across the chest. Stay off the soft tissue below the ribs.

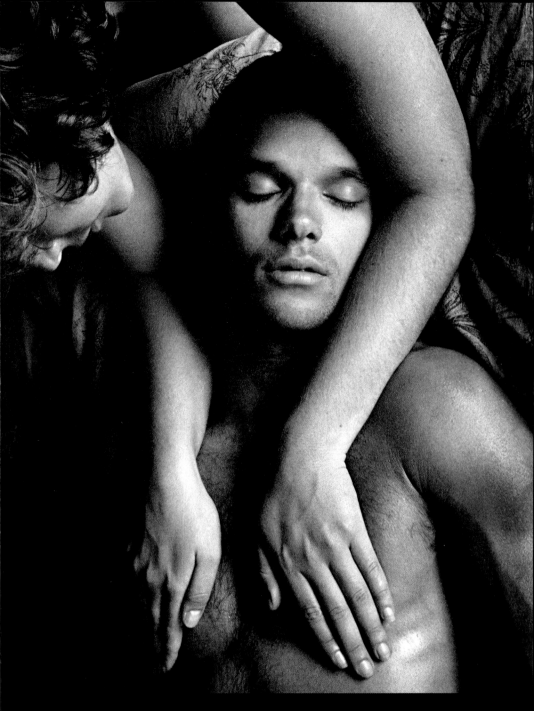

• Press the full, flat surface of your hands out from the center of the chest to the edge of the massage surface.

• Return to the starting point. Keep your contact pressure even throughout this stroke.

Reverse direction each time you reach the massage surface.

STROKING THE ABDOMEN

• Gently press your hands into the depression beneath the ribs and stroke forward and back. Turn your hand to the side as you descend. Focus on the full, flat surface of your palms as your hands glide past each other.

Abdominal muscles wrap
around the body.

KNEADING

• Knead from the hips to the armpits, using the full surface of your hand. Add oil as necessary.

• Use your thumb to pick up a fold of flesh with each cycle. Maintain the same rhythm up and down the side.

19

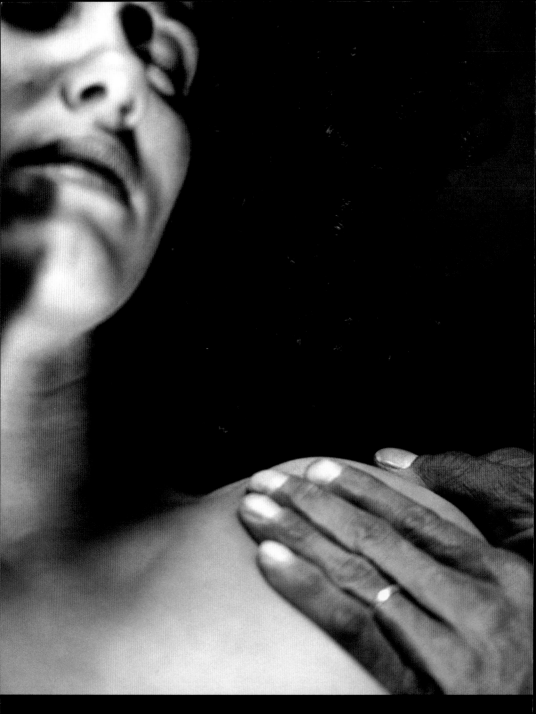

FINGERTIP FRICTION

- Anchor the stroke by sliding one hand beneath your partner's back and grasping the shoulder from below.
- Raise the shoulder slightly to meet your friction hand.
- Press down into the joint as you move in small, even circles.

Sensation zones are tied to spinal nerves.

HALF BODY STROKE

- Press the heels of your hands against your partner's shoulders with your fingers pointed toward the waist.
- Press forward. Then, turn and pull straight up from the waist, lifting the chest as you move toward the shoulders.

Your partner's chest will vibrate above your hands.

VIBRATING THE CHEST

- Sit at your partner's head and keeping your fingers pressed together, reach straight down below the shoulder blades.
- Lift straight up against the rib cage with your fingertips, pressing up and down in quick, short movements.

"I close my eyes and lose myself in the rubbing, while the fire, piled high, roars in the grate."
J.M. Coetzee, Waiting for the Barbarians

SWIMMING

• Begin with your thumbs touching at the center of the abdomen. Press forward with one hand while pulling back with the other, all the way to the massage surface at your partner's sides. Then return to the stomach.

23

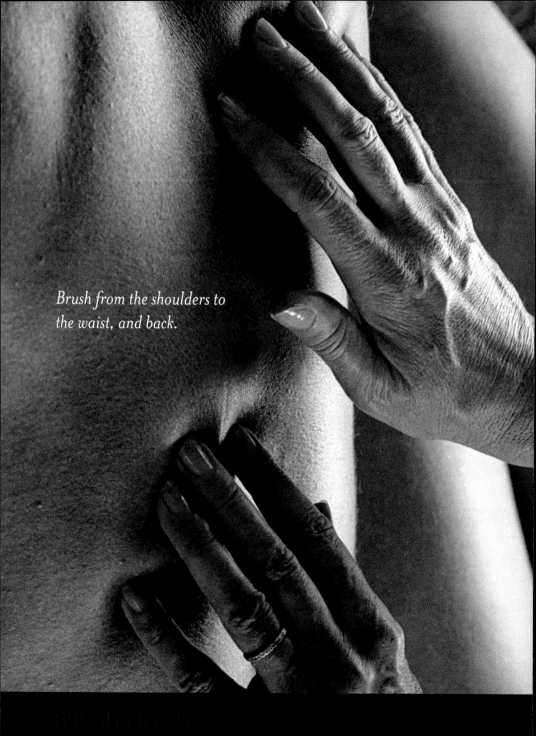

Brush from the shoulders to the waist, and back.

- Move sensation off the chest with your fingertips in a light hand-over-hand motion. Your partner will track the feeling.
- Vary the speed and length of your strokes. Break contact slowly at the shoulders.

HEAD

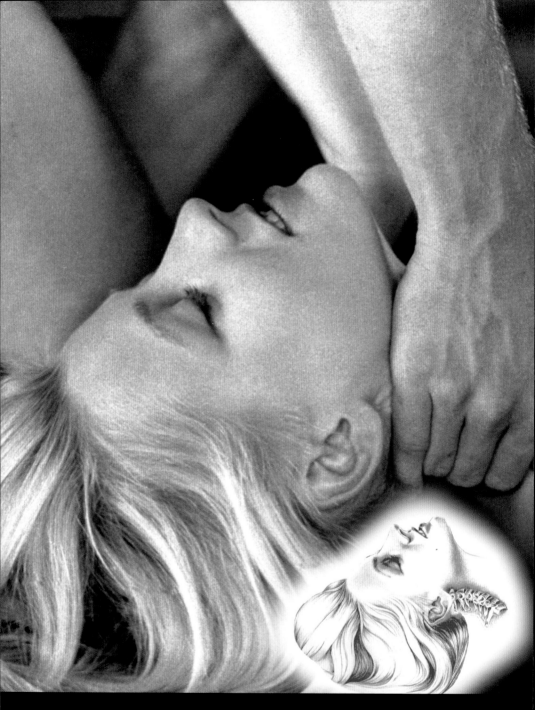

NECK LIFT

• Clasp your fingers basket-style just beneath your partner's neck and lift straight up. Move slowly. Avoid jerky motions.

• When you feel resistance, hold for a silent count of ten, before slowly lowering her neck.

Your hands make an invisible circle above your partners face.

STROKING THE FOREHEAD

- Cup your hands to make contact from temple to temple.
- Press forward with a light hand-over-hand motion on the forehead, lifting each hand as it passes over the eyes.
- As you lift one hand, maintain contact with the other.

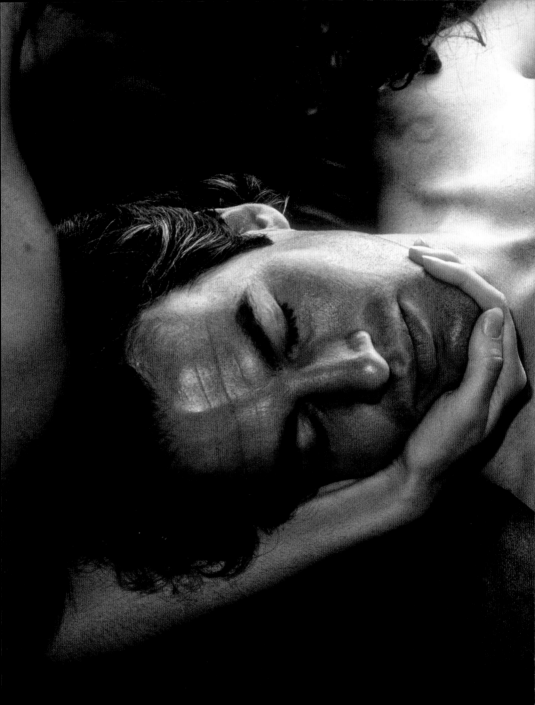

- Grasp the marked indentation at the base of the skull with one hand and your partner's chin with the other.
- Pull gently, straight backward, exerting equal pressure with both of your hands.

The eyelids have the thinnest skin on the body. Use very light pressure here, making contact only with the sides of your fingers.

STROKING THE EYES

- Anchor your thumbs on your partner's forehead and move your fingertips lightly across the top of his eyelids.
- Let your fingertips trace the depression just below the eyebrow. Reverse the stroke at the temples.

At 50, everyone has the face he deserves.
—*George Orwell*

As you massage the face, you will see stress-induced worry lines vanish as pure pleasure takes their place. That's one of the things human hands can do: erase stress lines.

STROKING THE FACE

- Pressing your palms against the sides of your partner's face, rotate slowly, first in the same, then in opposing directions.
- Make contact from the base of your hands to the fingertips.

Maintain pressure for about half a minute. Release it slowly.

PRESSING THE FOREHEAD

- Curve your hands to fit the precise contour of your partner's forehead. Press down evenly. Get feedback on pressure from your partner. Take your time. Let the feeling go on.

Placing your pinky over your partner's ear intensifies the tactile experience.

JAW FRICTION

- Press down lightly on the center of the forehead with your thumbs. Rotate your fingertips in small circles from the edge of the lips to the sides of the jaw—and face.
- Direct fingertip friction will relax the jaw and with it, the face.

*Think of the face as
a sensual palette.*

- With your thumbs raised (as shown) press up on the muscles at the back of your partner's neck.
- Rotate your fingers in opposing circles, with one hand up while the other is down. Stay off the spine itself.

Your partner will track the
sensation as it melts away.

PRESSING THE FACE

• Fold your hands over your partner's face, making contact from the base of your palms, on the cheeks, to the fingertips, over the scalp. Hold your contact for a silent count of ten and release it gradually.

Temple strokes can go on and on. Nobody ever objects.

CIRCLING THE TEMPLES

• Usually three or four fingertips will fit against the temples. Anchor with your thumbs over the center of the forehead. Pressing against the temples, rotate your fingertips in slow circles, three times in each direction.

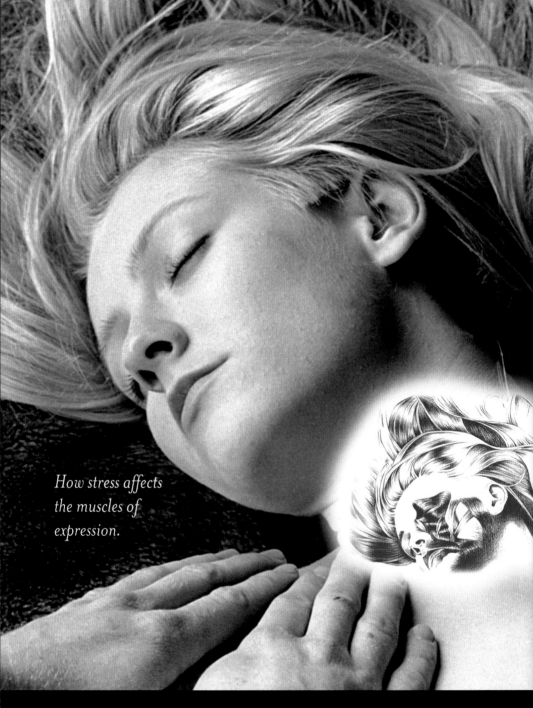

How stress affects the muscles of expression.

FINGERTIP FRICTION

- Tension is stored in the shoulders, scalp and jaws, but it registers first around the eyes and mouth.
- Rotate your fingertips on the the shoulders, then up the back of the neck to the jaw—and watch your partner's face relax.

ARMS

Press up the arm from wrist to shoulder.

CIRCULATION

- Cup your hands around your partner's wrist.
- Make contact from your fingertips to the base of your palms.
- Turn at the shoulder, allowing one hand to sweep over the top of the joint. Return to the wrists on the sides of the arm.

Add extra oil if necessary. Your hands should slide over, not pull at, the skin.

- Using the full flat surface of your hands, stroke out from the neck over both shoulders at once.
- Reverse the stroke at the top side of each arms.
- Bend your fingers around the shoulders as you stroke.

During massage, your partner's attention, usually focused on the world outside her body, becomes purely sensual; she follows your hands wherever they go.

FLEXING THE ARMS

- Anchor your partner's arm at the shoulder and pull back gently at the wrist. Turn the whole arm in sweeping circles, first in one direction then the other.
- If it's a first massage, get feedback on flexing pressure.

Need a break? Maintain contact (here, at the knee and wrist) while you rest.

FRICTION

- Anchor the shoulder with one hand and press the fingers of your other hand into the muscles that bend over the shoulder.
- Rotate slowly, moving back and forth on the muscular joint.

*Knead hand nerves from
the palm to the forearm.*

- Grasp the top of your partner's hand with your fingers while pressing inward against the palm with both thumbs.
- Rotate your thumbs—one up while the other is down.
- Use light pressure on the wrist and forearm.

Your thumbs should glide.
Add oil, if necessary.

KNEADING THE BICEPS

- Wrap your fingers around the arm and reach forward with the full, flat surface of your thumbs.
- Rotate the thumbs in opposing circles while pressing down into the muscular upper arm.

Squeeze the whole arm while it remains perfectly relaxed in a vertical position.

SQUEEZING THE ARM

• Lift the arm straight up at the wrist and squeeze gently.

• Squeeze and release with your fingers every few inches while moving from the shoulder to the wrist. Maintain a firm and consistent pressure up and down the arm.

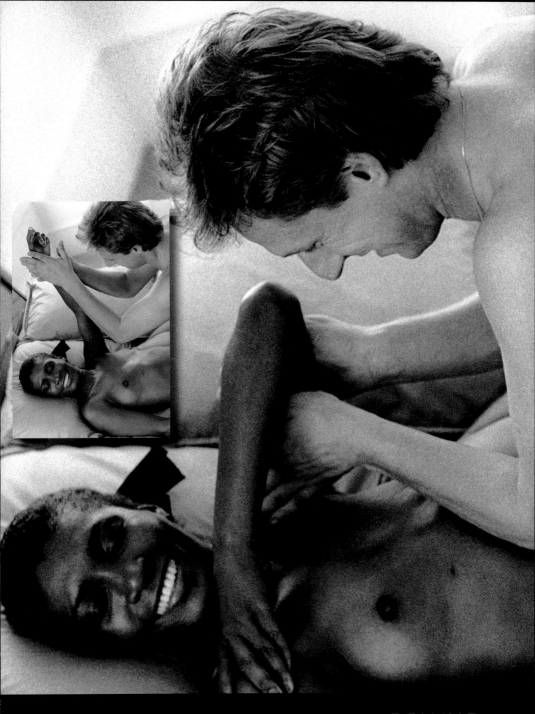

- Fold your partner's arm across her chest.
- With your fingers straight out, reach forward and grasp both sides of her upper arm close to the shoulder.
- Rock your hands back and forth as you move up the arm.

STRETCHING THE ARM

- Fold one hand over your partner's shoulder while pulling back on her opposite wrist.
- Stretch to the point of tension. Hold for a silent count of ten and release slowly.

*Kneading warms the whole shoulder and leaves
your partner basking in a warm, physical glow.*

KNEADING THE SHOULDERS

• Pick up a fold of flesh, with the fingers of one hand while the other hand opens wide. Circle as you knead.

• Press down into tight muscles with your fingertips as you knead. Use your full hand on muscular areas.

*Widen your circles a bit
as you repeat the stroke.*

ROTATING THE SHOLDER

• Kneel close to your partner and raise one knee for support. Use both hands to cup the shoulder from above and below (as shown). Rotate the whole joint making at least three comfortable circles in each direction.

HANDS

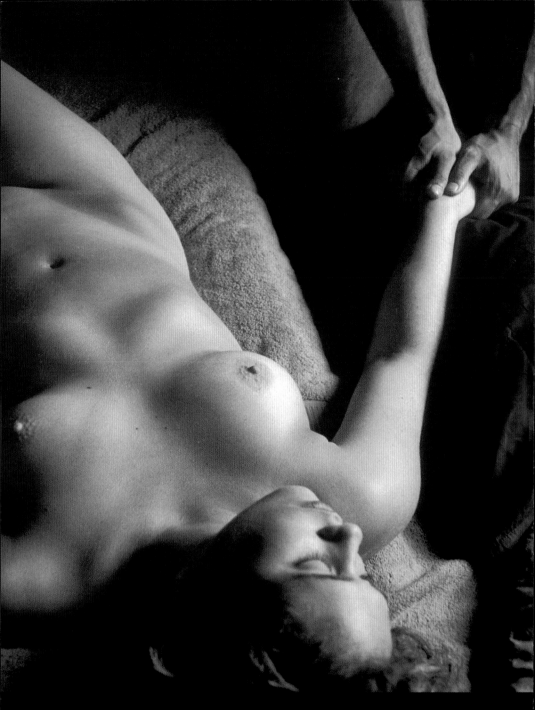

THUMB KNEADING

- Grip the palm side of your partner's hand using all four fingers of both your hands. Use less pressure with your thumbs than on the palm side.
- Rotate your thumbs, in small opposing circles.

Your partner's hand rotates just beneath the carpal ligament.

ROTATING THE HAND

• Anchor the arm just above the wrist and grasp your partner's fingers with your free hand.

• Rotate the hand in a rough circle, just inside the point of resistance. Turn three times in each direction.

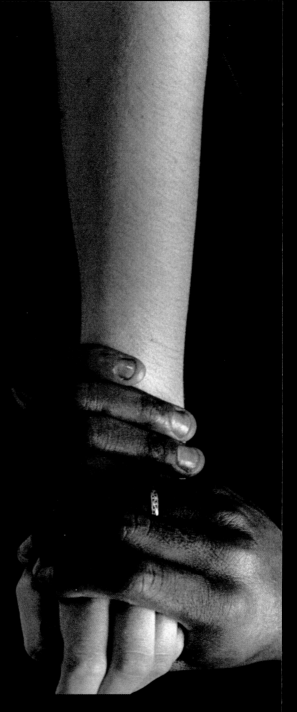

STROKING THE HAND

- Press forward across the wrist in short hand-over-hand strokes with one hand following close behind the other.
- Lift the front hand as soon as the back hand makes contact.

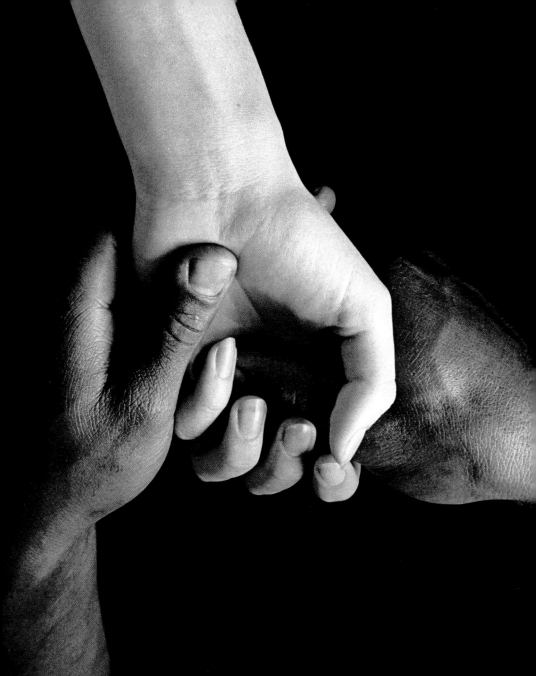

• Use both your hands to grasp the back of your partner's hand while pressing into the palm with both thumbs.

• Rotate your thumbs—one up, while the other is down—making small circles. Focus on the fleshy base of the palm.

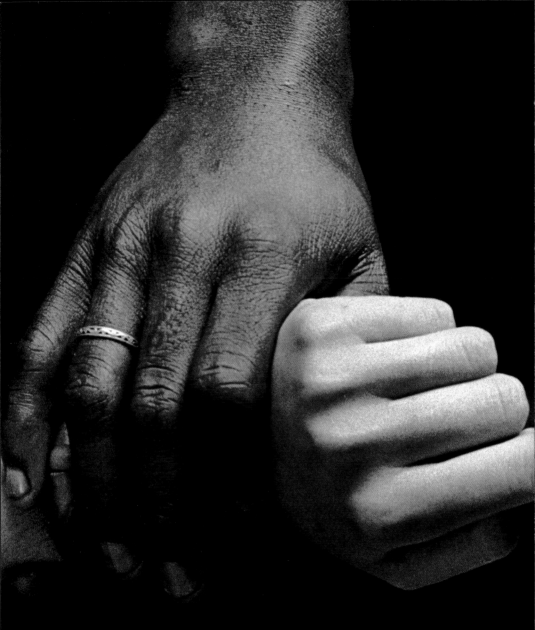

FLEXING THE WRIST

- Wrap your fingers around your partner's wrist. Pull gently toward the hand, maintaining the fully flexed position for a silent count of ten.
- As you release pressure gradually, the whole hand relaxes.

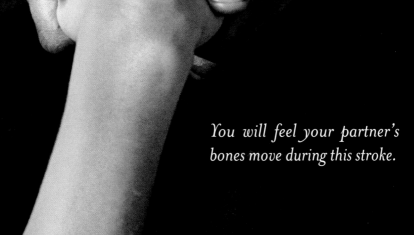

You will feel your partner's bones move during this stroke.

BONE ROLLING

• Squeeze your fingertips against your partner's palm. Gently rotate your hands in small circles, with one hand forward, while the other is back.

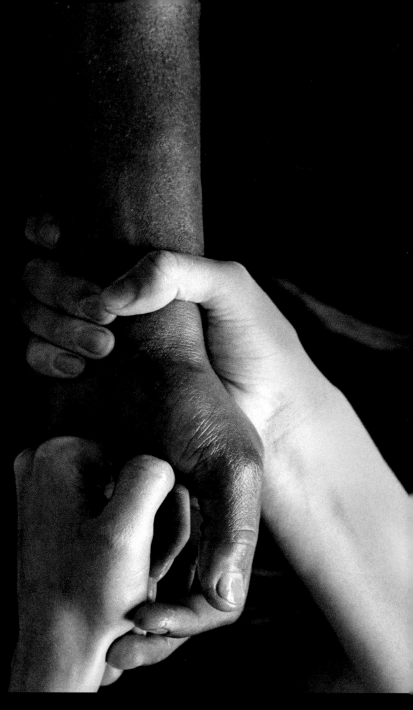

KNUCKLE PRESSING

- Grasp your partner's hand from below and press down into the palm with the flat surface of your knuckles.
- Rock your hand from side to side, then rotate it in small circles.

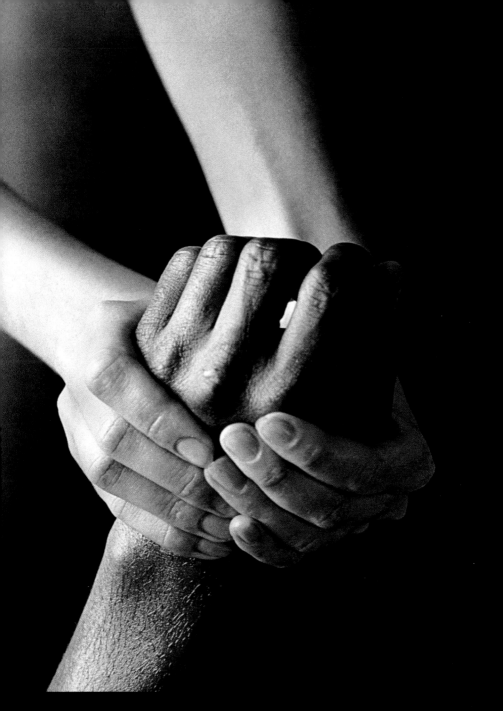

• Grasp the top of your partner's hand. Press up moderately hard against the palm with both thumbs.

• Pull outward with your clasped fingers from the center to the outside of the hand.

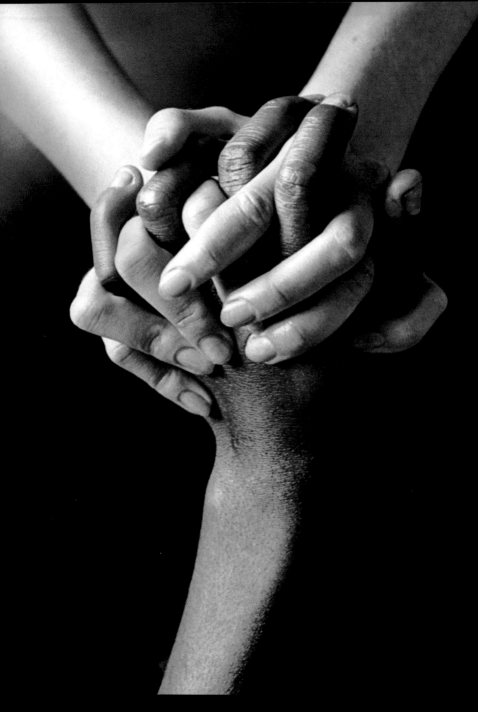

FLEXING THE FINGERS

- Weave all of your fingers between the fingers of your partner's hand—you decide what fits where—and gently bend the whole hand straight back at the wrist.
- Your hands seem to reach out for each other... and merge.

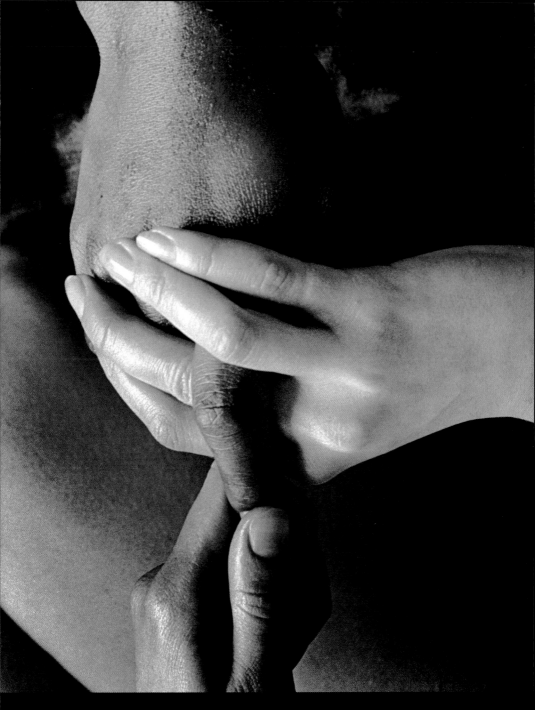

ROTATE THE FINGERS

• Grasp the tips of your partner's fingers one at a time and rotate three times in each direction. Maintain contact with your partner's hand as you move from one fingertip to another.

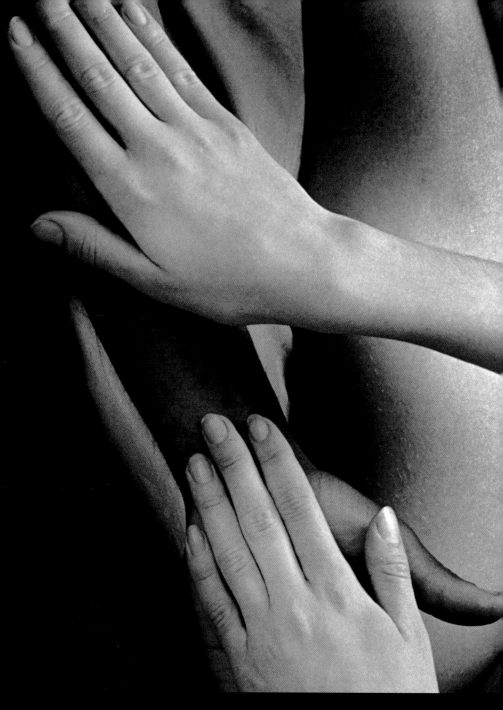

BRUSHING THE HAND

• Brush from the forearm to the fingertips in hand-over-hand strokes, some long, others short enough to focus on a single spot. Vary your brushing speed.

• Break contact slowly, fingertip to fingertip.

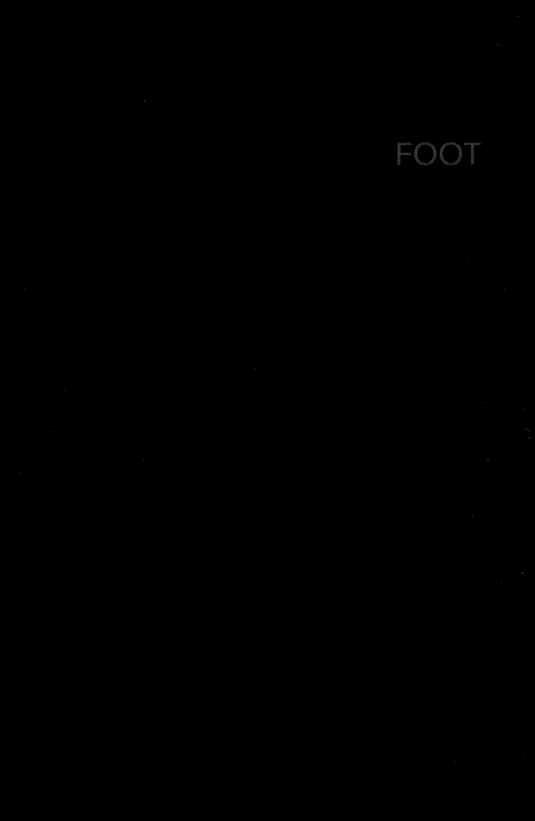

FOOT

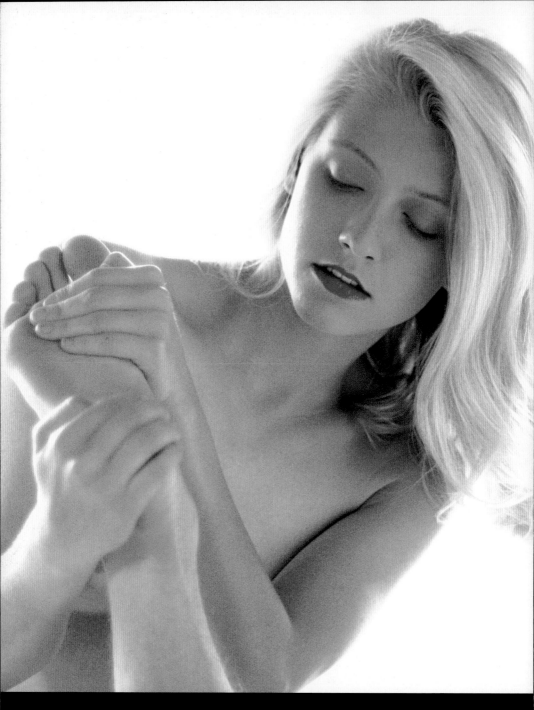

CIRCULATION

- Wrap your fingers over the bottom of the foot.
- Press forward, over the heel to the ankle. Return along the sides of the foot to your starting position.
- Vary your speed and end above the ankle on the calf.

Listen: soft moaning means you've got it right.

PRESSING THE ARCH

- Press down into the arch with the flat part of your knuckles.
- Support the foot from below while you press down.
- The bottom of the foot will accept more pressure than any other part of the body.

"And after she had bathed him and anointed him with olive oil, and cast about him a goodly mantle, he came forth from the bath in fashion like the deathless Gods."
The Odyssey, Homer

KNEADING THE SOLE

- Grasp the top of the foot with all four fingers of each hand.
- Press down into the center of the arch with your thumbs.
- Keep the thumbs close to each other as you circle.

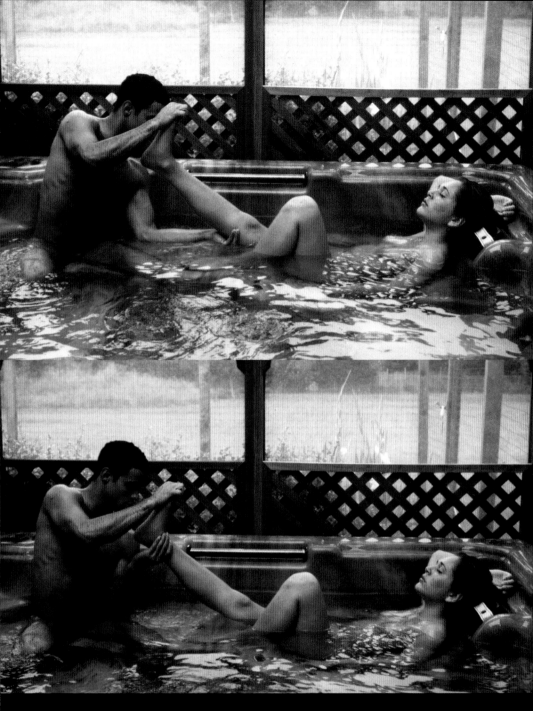

- Lift your partner's leg above the knee and at the ankle.
- While supporting her leg above the knee, gently bend her foot forward and back at the toes.
- Support the leg at the ankle and knee as you lower it.

*The large tibial nerve
ends on the arch.*

CIRCLING THE ARCH

- Grasp the top of the foot with one hand while circling on your partner's arch with the fingertips of the other.
- Use the full flat surface of your fingertips.

As you knead, maintain an even rhythm with both thumbs.

KNEADING THE FOOT

- Wrap your fingers around your partner's heel and circle with the flat surfaces of your thumbs.
- Move from the back of the ankle to the bottom of the foot.
- Press down hard on the arch.

FOOT ROTATION

- Lift and support your partner's ankle with one hand while grasping the foot below the toes with your other hand.
- Rotate the top of the foot in small circles.

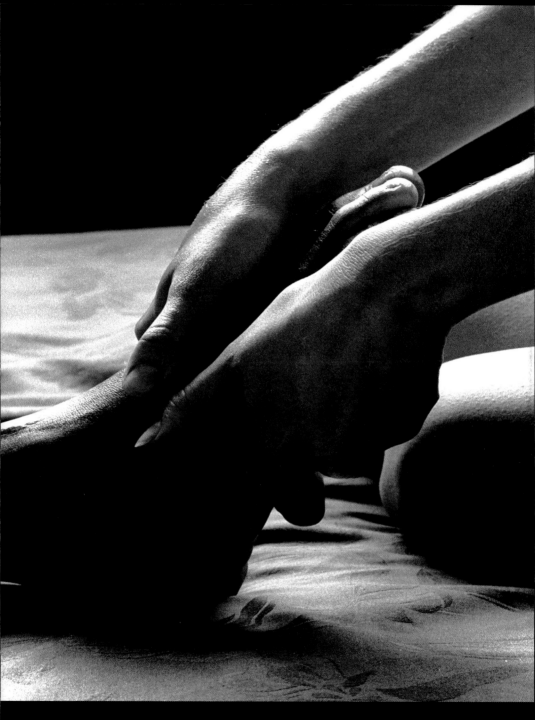

KNEADING THE FOOT

- Grasp the bottom of the foot with all four fingers and knead the top with your thumbs. Press down with the full, flat surface of your thumb, making generous circles in each direction.
- Knead from the ankle to the the toes and back.

This simple pulling motion will be felt halfway across the body as joints at the ankle, knee and hip flex together.

LEG STRETCH

- Grasp the heel with one hand and wrap your other hand across the top of the foot.
- Pull back equally at the heel and the top of the foot.
- Hold at the point of resistance for a silent count of ten.

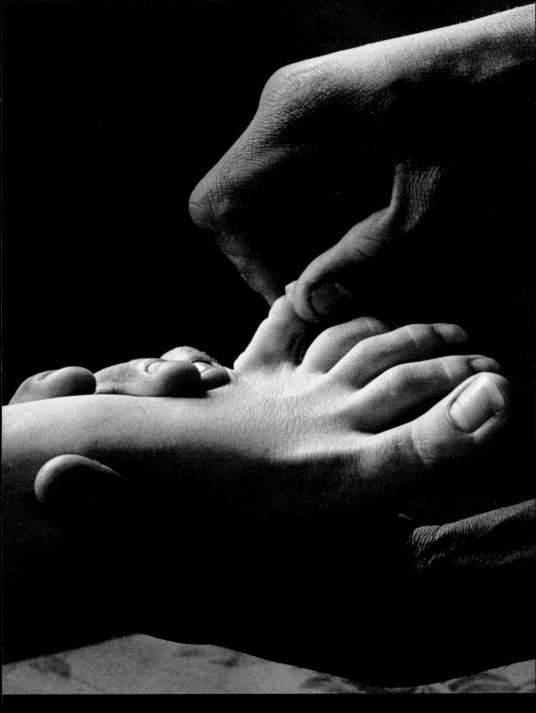

TOE PLAY

- Pull down the sides of each toe in a corkscrew motion, twisting your fingers in a half circle from the bottom of the toe to the top.
- Grasp the end of each toe and rotate it in each direction.
- Fold your hand over the toes and flex them gently.

*Break contact slowly
at the tips of the toes.*

BRUSHING THE FOOT

- Brush down the leg with your fingertips from the hips.
- Moving down in a hand-over-hand motion, cover the legs with long and short strokes. Increase speed on the foot, ending with rapid strokes from the ankle to the toes.

FRONT OF THE LEGS

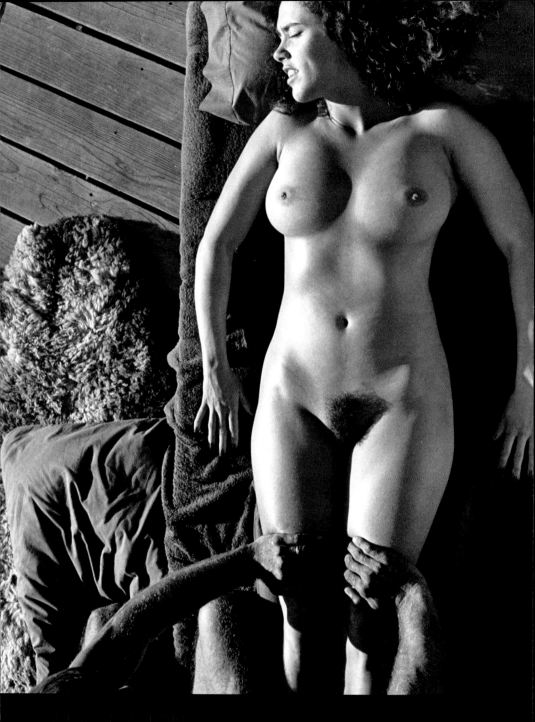

- Cup your fingers around the calf, keeping your left hand on top on the right leg, your right hand on top on the left leg.
- Turn at the hips. Return to the ankle on the side of the leg, making light contact.

Vary the stroke by lifting with both hands below the knees (as shown).

ROTATING THE LEGS

- Support your partner's leg above and below the knee and lift to the point of resistance.
- Stretch the leg back gently several times, then lower it slowly to the massage surface.

75

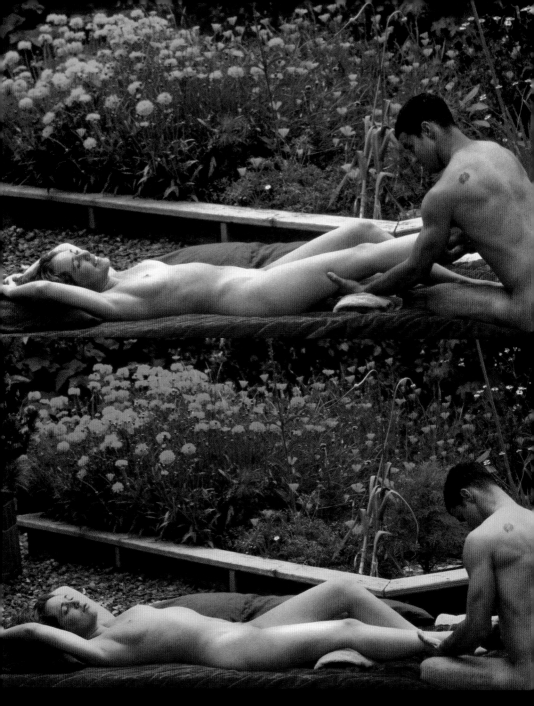

STROKING THE CALF

- Wrap your hands around the back of the thigh and calf, making contact from the base of your palms to the tips of your fingers.
- Pull hand-over-hand to the foot, moving from the knee to the ankle. Vary your speed as you repeat the stroke.

A few seconds of very quick stroking spreads penetrating warmth.

FAST KNEE STROKING

- Raise your partner's legs to bring the knees to a bent position.
- Keeping your fingers pressed together, move your hands back and forth against the side of each knee.

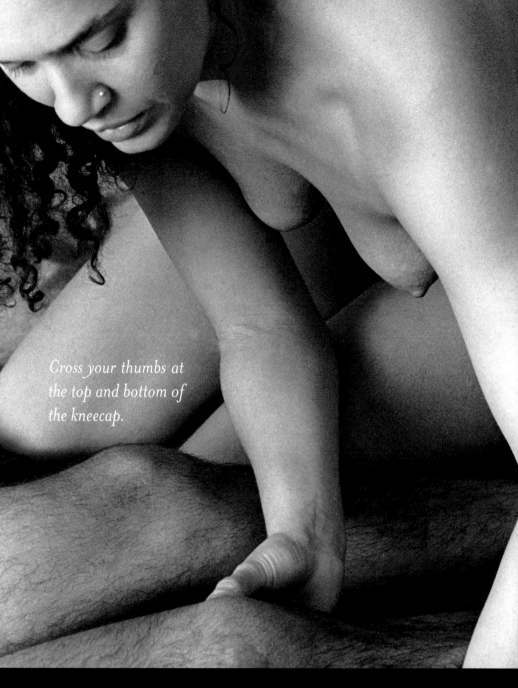

Cross your thumbs at the top and bottom of the kneecap.

CIRCLING THE KNEE

- Tucking your thumbs under the kneecap, wrap your other fingers around the back of the knee.
- Circle the knee three times in each direction with your thumbs, pressing inward as you go.

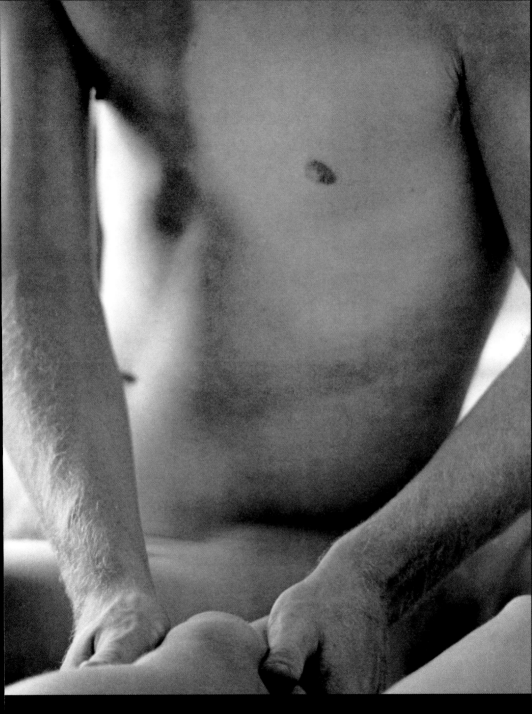

FINGERTIP KNEADING

- Folding your fingers around the bottom of the leg, reach forward with your thumbs.
- Rotate the tips of your thumbs in opposing circles starting just below the kneecap and moving down to the top of the foot.

*Forearm meets calf—when was the
last time that happened for you?*

THE CALF TWIST

- Oil your forearm. Kneel at your partner's foot and raise her leg to relax the calf muscles.
- Anchor her leg at the ankle while rotating your forearm against her calf. Move from ankle to knee and back.

*Rotate your hands in tight
circles while you knead.*

• Reach across your partner's body and knead up the leg from the ankle, picking up a fold of flesh with one hand while the other opens wide. Use your thumbs to pick up flesh, squeezing gently and then releasing.

81

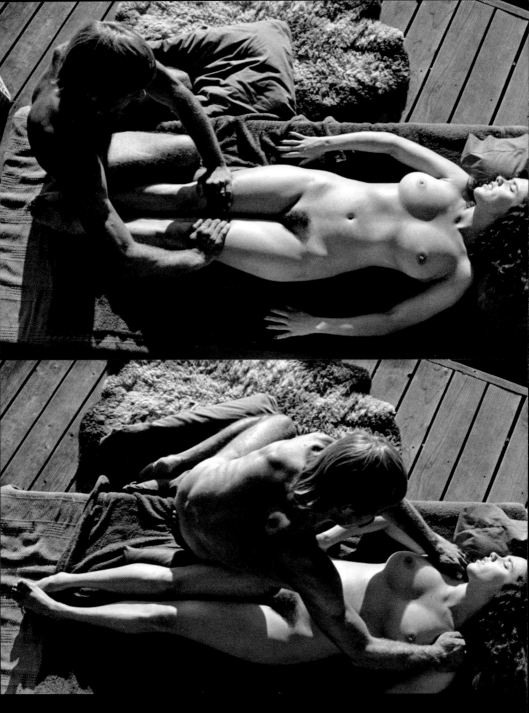

BODY CIRCULATION

- Oil the front and sides of your partner's legs and chest.
- Wrap your palms around the sides of the ankles and press up the legs letting your hands flatten out on the chest.
- Move back down the sides of the body to the ankles.

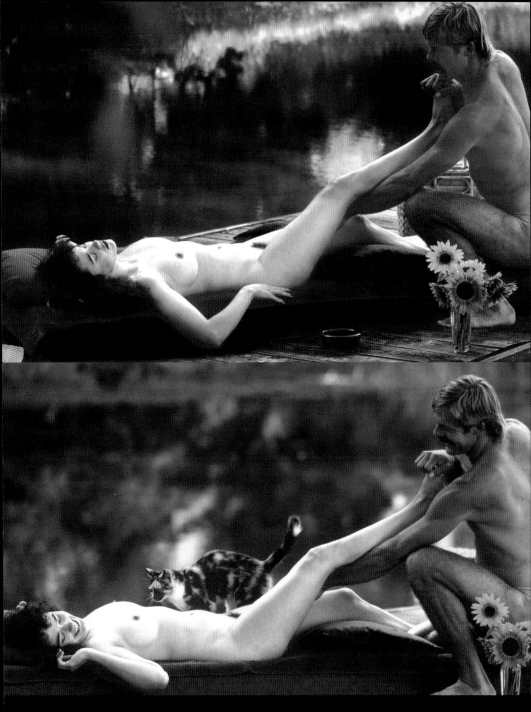

FLEXING THE CALF

- Balance your body tripod-style, with one knee up and the other down. Grasp the inside of your partner's thigh (as shown). Lift the top of the foot with your free hand.
- Bend the foot forward at the toes while rotating the leg.

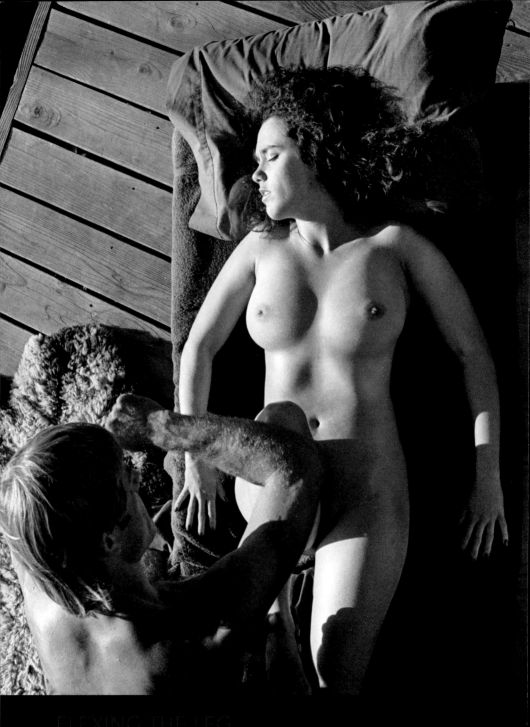

FLEXING THE LEG

- Grasp the ankle and press forward on the knee with the inside of your forearm.
- Push to the point of resistance, hold for a moment and release slowly. Bring the leg and foot down. Then flex the other leg.

BACK

THE BACK LIFT

- Reach under the armpits and clasp your hands behind your partner's neck. Lift slowly, to the point of resistance, avoiding sharp jerky motions.
- Hold the top of your partner's body, suspended in air.

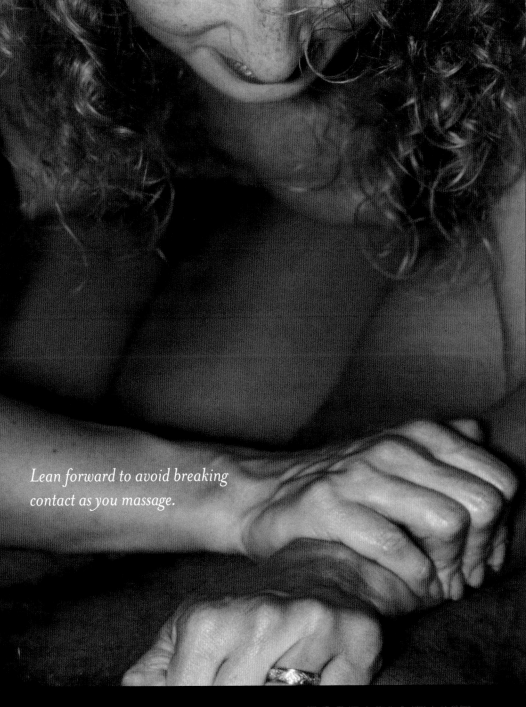

Lean forward to avoid breaking contact as you massage.

- Reach across your partner's spine and twist on the opposite side of his back. Make contact from the flat part of your knuckles to the fleshy inner forearm. Turn your whole forearm in generous circles, pressing down as you move up and down the back.

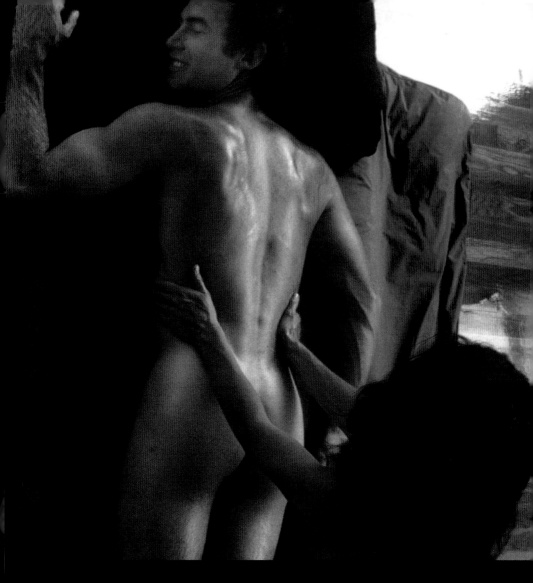

- To reach both the shoulders and feet, kneel above your partner's knee. Oil the back from the waist to the shoulders, making sure to include the sides as well.

- Flatten your hands at your partner's hips so the spine passes between your thumbs.

- Press up to the shoulders on the muscular ridges that run parallel to the spine, staying off the spine itself.

- Turn across the shoulders, making contact from the fingertips to the base of your palms.

• Return down the sides of the body to your starting point.

*Turn just inside the point
where you feel tension.*

- Anchor the shoulder from below with one hand and press down from above with the other.
- Lean forward and lift the whole shoulder.
- Rotate slowly, keeping a firm grip on both sides.

Reverse the stroke, pulling back at the shoulder while pushing forward at the hip.

FLEXING THE BACK

- Pull back with your elbow while pressing forward with the heel of your hand. Bend gently to the point of tension.
- Then, bend your elbow over the front of your partner's hip while folding your hand over the back of her shoulder.

FLEXING THE SHOULDERS

- Cup one hand over your partner's shoulder, pulling back on her other shoulder with your folded arm.
- Press gently to the point of tension and release slowly. Then, reverse the stroke, pressing forward where you pulled back.

Spend extra time on visible muscles.

ELBOW TAPPING

- The tip of your elbow fits nicely over the long muscles that run parallel to your partner's spine.
- Strike your palm while guiding your elbow tip along muscled portions of the back. Stay off the spine.

Knead up and down the long muscles on the side of the body.

KNEADING

- Move your hands in opposing circles, picking up a fold of flesh with the fingertips of one hand, while releasing one with the other. Maintain an even rhythm up and down the side.
- Knead from the shoulder to the side of the knee and return.

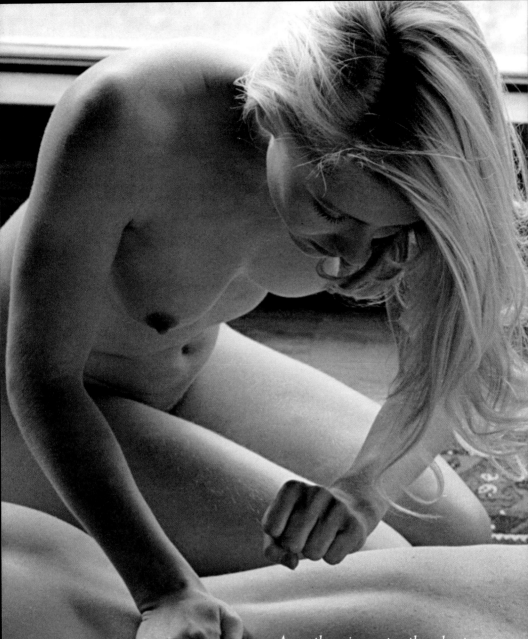

A gentle rain, not a thunderstorm.
Keep it up for a while; make it last.

PERCUSSION

- Bending each percussion hand at the wrist before you make contact absorbs the force of the impact.
- Your partner feels a light, exhilarating tapping that travels up and down the back.

Thumb kneading travels well.
Try it on the legs.

THUMB PRESSING

• Open one hand wide and pick up a fold of flesh with the thumb of your other hand. Press forward.
• Rotate your thumb in small circles on the muscular parts of your partner's back.

Push down on the muscles below and rotate your fingertips.

SPOT FRICTION

• Anchor above or below the massage area, using the whole surface of one hand with your thumb spread wide.

• Press into the area between thumb and forefinger with all four fingers of your other hand. Maintain pressure, while rotating.

BACK OF THE LEGS

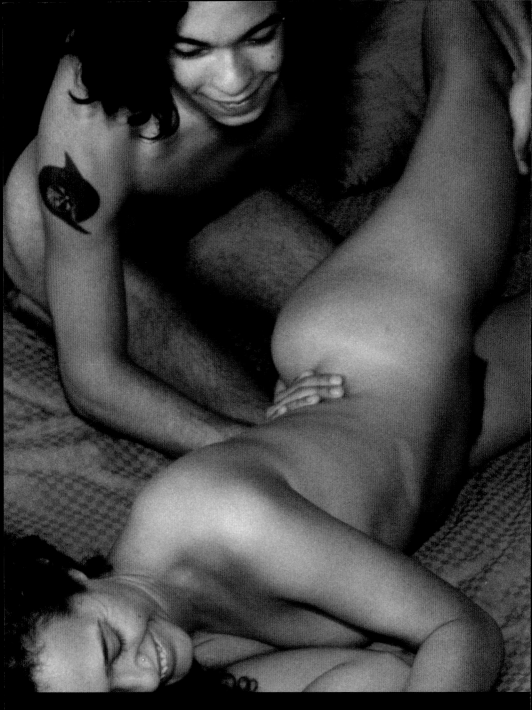

THE HIP ROLL

- Stabilize your partner's leg above the knee with one hand while pressing the small of the back with the other.
- Lift her leg to the point of resistance. Her body will remain still while the hip stretches luxuriously.

Move back to the ankle on the side of the leg, making light contact on your return stroke.

CIRCULATION

- Cup your fingers over the muscular calf.
- Move back, leading with your right hand on the left leg and your left hand on the right leg.
- Press forward to the hips, turning at the buttocks.

Massage is applied kindness. It's a tangible gift of pleasure and it costs nothing if you do it yourself.

FLEXING THE KNEE

- Anchor by steadying the back of the knee with one hand while you bend your partner's leg toward his hip.
- Keep your anchor hand in place on the return.

Add enough oil to make your hands glide.

STROKING THE BACK OF THE LEGS

• Wrapping your fingers around the leg, stroke down from the thigh to the ankle with one hand, then the other.

• Vary your speed on the descent moving from long, slow strokes to moderately fast short repetitions. A thriller.

Press to the point of tension and release gradually.

FLEXING THE HIPS

- Pull back across your partner's hip with the side of your elbow, while pressing forward on the shoulder with your free hand.
- Then, push the hip forward with the heel of your hand and pull back at the shoulder with the side of your elbow.

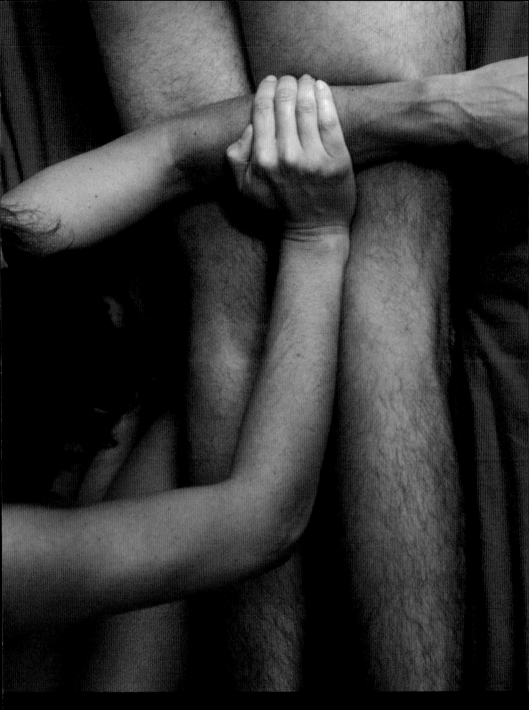

- Grasp your arm directly over your partner's thigh. Press down while circling slowly. Vary the stroke by reaching across the legs and rotating on both legs at once.
- Move from the thighs to the ankles and back.

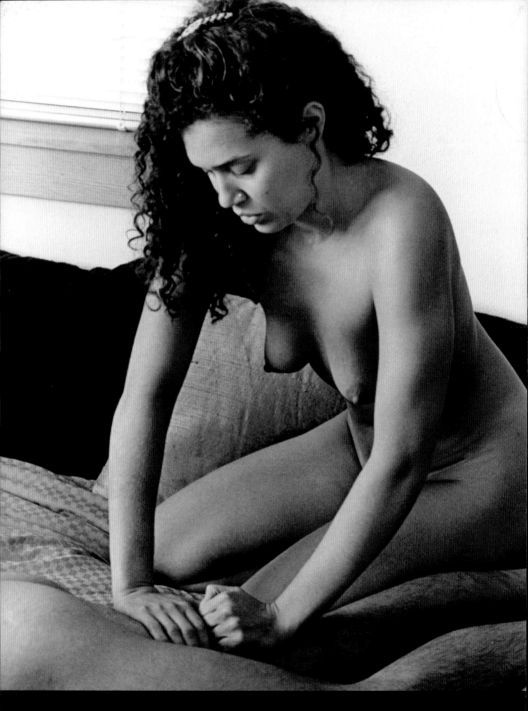

DEEP FRICTION

• Anchor the stroke with one hand and make a fist with the other. Press down with the flat part of your knuckles until you feel solid muscle. Reduce pressure on the back of the knee to spare close-to-the surface blood vessels.

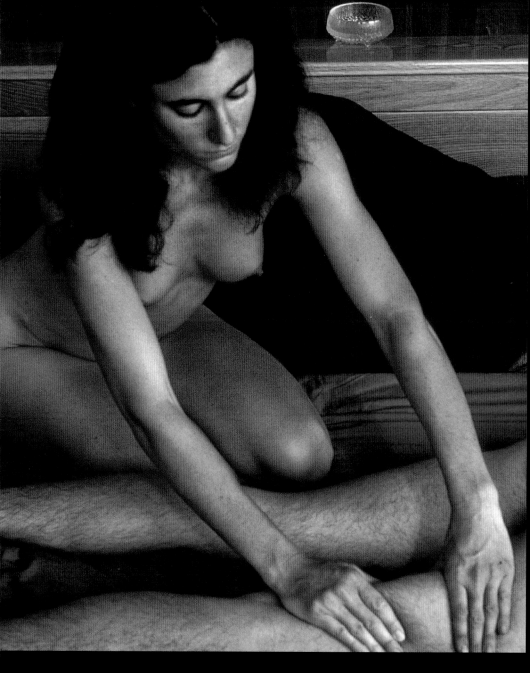

KNEADING

• Reach across your partner's body and knead up the leg from the ankle, picking up a fold of flesh with one hand while the other opens wide. Use your thumbs to pick up flesh, squeezing gently and then releasing.

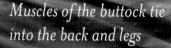

*Muscles of the buttock tie
into the back and legs*

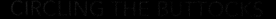

CIRCLING THE BUTTOCKS

• Press down evenly so the full flat surface of your hands grips your partner's skin.

• As you turn your hands in gentle opposing circles—one hand up, the other down—your partner's buttocks will rotate slowly.

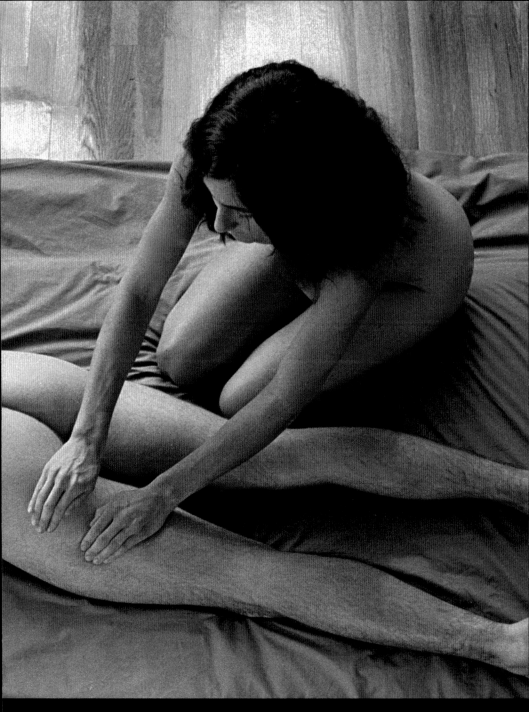

PERCUSSION

- Clap up and down the leg, keeping your hands cupped.
- Bend your hands at the wrists to cushion the impact.
- Keep your hands close together, thumbs brushing each other occasionally, as you travel up and down the leg.

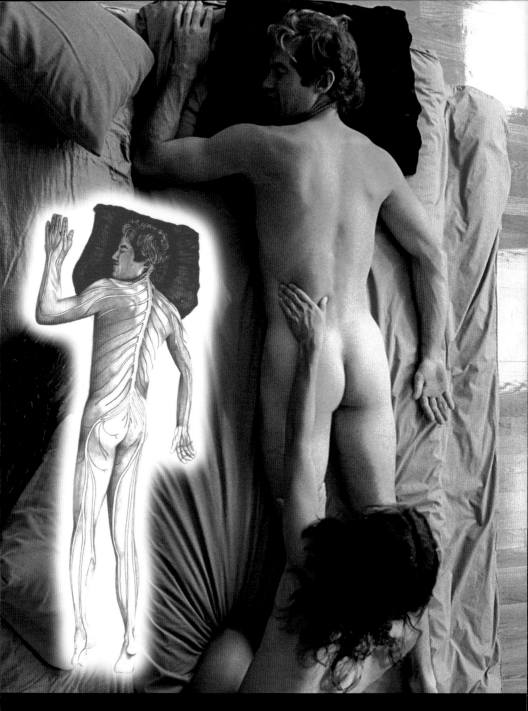

BRUSHING THE LEGS

- Brush the back of the legs from the hips to the toes with your full hand, then with your fingertips.
- Mix long and short strokes.
- End at the ankles or toes and move on to back massage.

SPECIALTIES

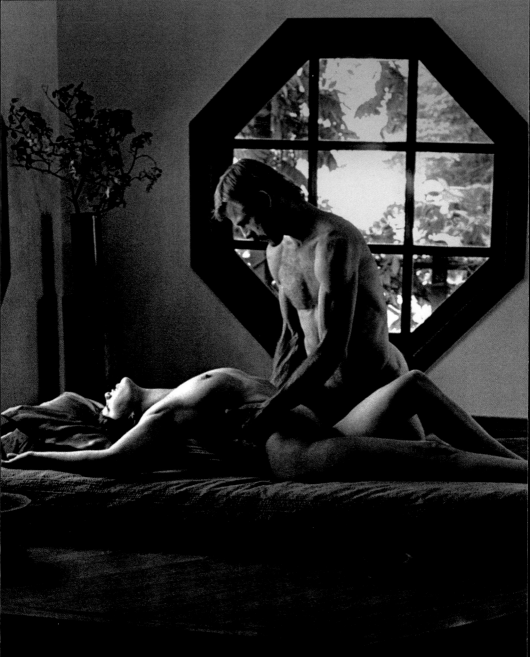

THE MASSAGE GIFT

- Celebrate your next special occasion by giving a massage.
- Think of a gift massage as a kind of pleasure snapshot, which your partner will recall for years afterwards.
- This time you will be there to share the pleasure with her.

"All lovers swear more performance than they are able,
and yet reserve an ability that they never perform…"
Troilus and Cressida, William Shakespeare

• Erotic massage turns sex into a sensual feast. If ever mind and body will merge for your partner, they will do so now.
• if you are searching for an aphrodisiac, a way to ignite your sex life, try massage.

Use massage to awaken the neglected 90% of the body: the feet, the sides of the knees and the shoulders.

EROTIC

- How many lovers have confined their touching to the so called "erogenous zones," a mere 5 or 10% of the body?
- If you have been searching for an aphrodisiac, a way to ignite your sex life, try sensual massage.

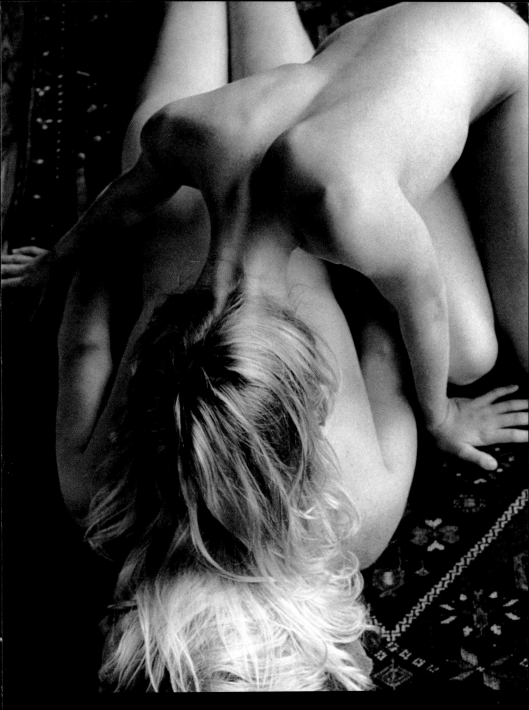

- With this single stroke, your partner will get the point of sensual massage—and you will get the credit.
- Lower your head until your forehead is nearly parallel with your partner's body. Move up and down the body.

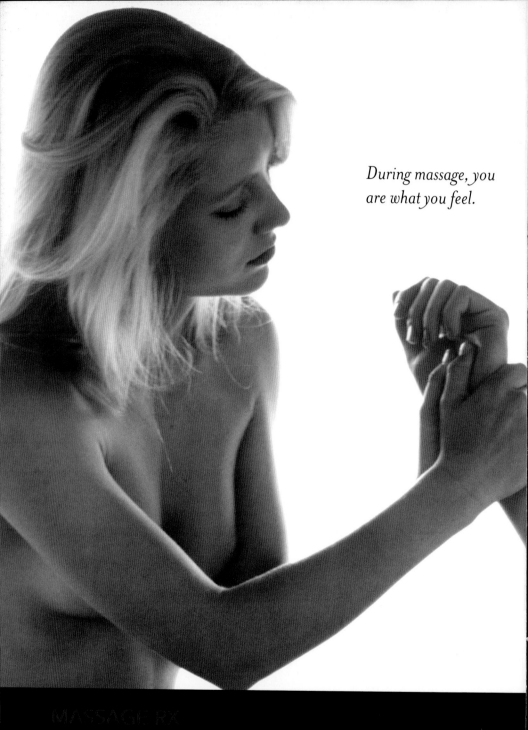

During massage, you are what you feel.

- Nervous? Most anxieties are inventions of the mind.
- By animating the tactile sense, massage thrusts your partner into the here and now.
- Massage reduces anxiety by relaxing the body.

Five people, ten hands, fifty fingers.

GROUP

• Not one person in 10,000 has been massaged by 5 people at once. That's simply got to change.

• It seems difficult to believe that anything in life could possibly be more wonderful.

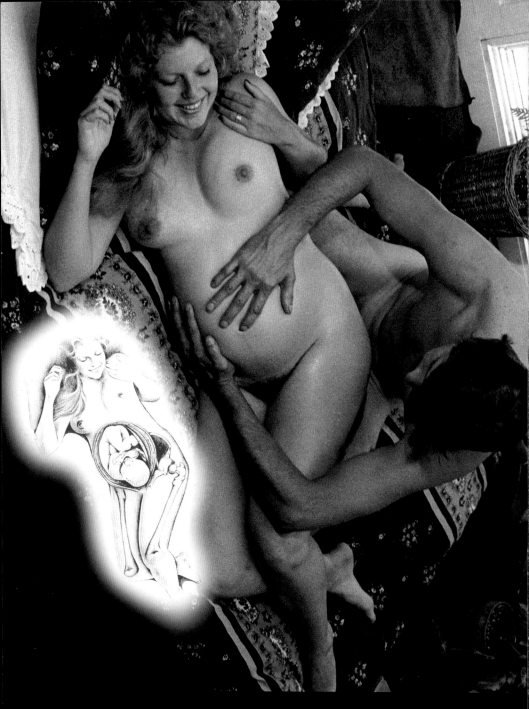

PREGNANCY

• Massage provides a practical role for the father-to-be.

• Daily massage will add, tangibly, to the expectant mother's sense of well-being. And it brings a wonderful new skill into the family: the ability to give pleasure with your hands.

Don't speak. Words will come between your partner and the feeling. Let your hands say it.

TWILIGHT

- As you learn massage try lowering the lights.
- Your partner will have his eyes closed.
- As light is reduced, tactile sensations are amplified.

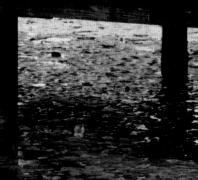

After an hour of sensual massage your partner will have trouble remembering what she was stressed about.

STRESS CONTROL

• Masseurs see stress as a physical, not an emotional, issue and work on it through the body. Irritating acidic wastes are stored in tensed muscles. Relax the muscles and the wastes are dispersed. During massage peace becomes a tangible sensation.

Books:

The Art of Sensual Massage

Sensual Massage for Couples

Massage for a Peaceful Pregnancy

Super Massage

The New Sensual Massage

Ergonomic Living (with Iris Schencke)

Videos:

The Art of Sensual Massage

Classic Stars of Bellydance

SENSUAL MASSAGE
Made Simple ™

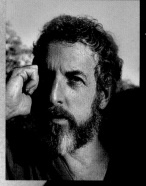

Written and Photographed by
Gordon Inkeles

Cover and Art Direction: Rama Wong
Layout and Photo Editing: Scott Harrison
Matching Anatomical Illustrations: Sigga Bjornsson
Production Assistant: Taavi Taijala
Author Photo: C.I. Schencke

ABOUT THE AUTHOR

Gordon Inkeles' bestselling books and DVDs (sensualmassage.net) have become standard reference works on massage throughout the world. His work has been translated into ten languages and reprinted more than sixty times. His book "The Art of Sensual Massage" has sold over one million copies. His film "The Art of Sensual Massage" played to SRO crowds at the Cannes Film Festival. Internationally known as a college lecturer and leader of massage workshops, Inkeles lives with his family in Northern California.